Dear Friend,

I must admit, I was at my wits end trying to figure out where these painful red bumps were coming from. Some of them looked like pimples while others were just a pin-head size bump. I have to confess, I tried to pop a few of the larger red bumps with *white "heads"* on the top with no success. I seem to only *"anger" my skin* like a volcano ready to erupt but wanting to terrorize the local area for as long as possible. *My skin was hot, red, blotch, dry and extremely itchy* in patches here and there and in places I'd rather not mention.

I thought I could "fix" my skin myself andtried lots of over-the-counter lotions. You can probably imagine what came to pass with those…some of them did *nothing* while others made my skin condition *worse than ever*. I *became self-conscious* about my skin and the way I looked; the itching was unbearable at times. I began wearing long-sleeves and pants in the summer. I wanted to *wear a veil over my face* but decided to go to a dermatologist instead.

The first dermatologist was young and after a hasty look from across the room – as if I were contagious – she stated she had never seen my condition before, which was not exact reassuring. She left the room and I'm sure merely "Googled" red skin bumps before returning with my diagnosis. She claimed I had *"hot tub folliculitis"* or maybe *"barber's itch"*. When I asked for an explanation, she basically told me not to worry, that it would *"go away on its own" in a few days*. I politely explained that I had not been in a hot tub in over 20 years and never stepped foot in a barber shop. And unless whatever "it" was could "leap" off my husband, who does frequent a barber, then she was *incorrect with her diagnosis*. Plus, I had this condition for several months now. I should have *kept my mouth shut*. No doctor, even relatively new ones like to be told they are wrong. She handed me a few sample packets of an antibacterial cream and I left, even more ashamed.

After about a week of more itching, increasing sadness and growing shame, I decided *I had to do something*. I was not going to leave *my skin, my health* up to someone else, someone who did not know how to *treat me with respect*. Even if this young doctor did have the right answers for my skin condition, she was sorely lacking in her people skills.

I used the two terms she provided me with: *"hot tub folliculitis"* and *"barber's itch"* and began searching the Internet for everything I could find about these and other skin conditions that could be causing my painful, red rashy skin. Once I discovered **what** I had, I continued to search for **how** to cure it. ***Folliculitis is a painful skin infection*** and if not treated properly can become devastating to other parts of the body.

I'm here to tell you**, *there is hope***. There is no reason to suffer through hot summers with long-sleeves or stay inside in shame because of your skin. And scratching yourself to a bloody mess is not the answer either. ***Folliculitis*** is more common than people realize and ***you can have clear, bump-free skin once again***.

I want to share the ***information and treatments that helped me clear my folliculitis*** so that others do not have to go through the pain, suffering and embarrassment I went through. Knowledge and awareness is vital to discovering the best way back to ***clear, itch-free skin***. I hope what I have learned on my way to beautiful skin benefits you on your journey to better skin and overall health as well.

Best regards,

Table of Contents

Preventing Folliculitis

Final Thoughts

The Many Faces of Folliculitis

There are several types of the skin problems, which are listed under the main category folliculitis. Folliculitis happens when damage occurs in the hair follicles. The damage could be from clothing friction (rubbing), a blocked follicle or shaving. Bacteria and fungus are two issues that cause folliculitis and are described as small red bumps, some with a "whitehead" that are similar to pimples and can be very painful in some individuals. Shaving, plucking and improper hygiene can be contributing factors to another type of folliculitis that also shows up as red, itchy blistery and pimply looking bumps on the surface of the skin. Ingrown hairs, something you may feel you have little control over, is yet another cause of a subcategory of folliculitis.

The two central types of folliculitis skin conditions are superficial folliculitis and deep folliculitis. Superficial folliculitis is often mildly itchy but not unbearable and will more often than not, clear up without intervention. Deep folliculitis is the severe form of the two skin conditions. Deep folliculitis is painful and often requires a visit to your healthcare provider or dermatologist.

Unfortunately, even with modern medication prescribed by your doctor, this itchy, painful and often embarrassing skin condition could keep returning, leaving both visible scars and deep tissue scars. There is a laser treatment for folliculitis which has seen some success in some individuals. But this type of treatment is typically expensive and insurance companies are not always willing to pay for laser treatments.

There are several homeopathic remedies for folliculitis which many individuals have reported experiencing great success with. But prevention is also a key component for curing and then maintaining clear, beautiful and healthy skin.

Types of Folliculitis

When one or more hair follicles become inflamed, you are at risk of developing folliculitis. Since your entire body is covered in skin, as well as tiny pores or follicles where hair grows from, you can develop folliculitis anywhere on your body. Some hairs are so thin, so fine; you may not even notice them until they become infected.

What is a Hair Follicle?

A hair follicle is defined as being a very small opening, sometimes as small as a pin-hole or smaller, in the skin's surface. Under the surface, the follicle is a long, narrow cylindrical shape. This cylinder form holds a number of layers, each with a different job to perform in order to keep the hair growing and looking good, in the case of hair on your head. Located at the base, inside each hair follicle, is a protrusion or stick-type projectile known as the papilla. The papilla contains many tiny blood vessels or capillaries that feed the cells within each hair strand growing out of every follicle.

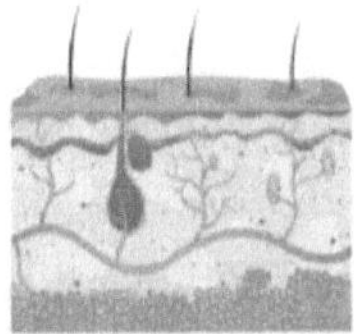

The part of the hair that is living is at the lowermost portion of the cylindrical shape. This is called the bulb and it is covered by papilla. It is also the only part which is fed by capillaries. According to cell research, the cells contained within the hair follicle bulb will divide every 23 to 72 hours, which is faster than cells located in any other part of the human body.

Gram-negative Folliculitis – When an individual is on a long-term antibiotic, commonly prescribed for the treatment of acne, Gram-negative Folliculitis can develop on different parts of their body, sometimes on or near the area of acne originally being treated. The balance of normal bacteria located in the nose, is often altered by antibiotics with the result an overgrowth of Gram-negative, the harmful bacteria. Typically, this does not bother people and when they finish the antibiotics and their nose flora returns to normal. However, there are some individuals in which the Gram-negative bacterium spreads beyond the nasal passages to cause additional, hard-to-treat acne lacerations.

SycosisBarbae Folliculitis – This type of deep folliculitis often come about in young men who recently began shaving. In this particular folliculitis skin condition, the entire hair follicle becomes inflamed and tiny pustules appear around the upper lip, the chin and jawline. The pustules become enlarged as the years spent shaving continues. Severe cases of Sycosis Barbae Folliculitis could leave scars.

Eosinophilic Folliculitis – This type of deep folliculitis is largely seen in patients with HIV and found on their upper arms, face or back. Eosinophilic folliculitis is inflamed, red sores and some are filled with white or yellow pus. These patches of sores are intensely itchy and when they heal, will leave the skin darker than it normally was. Why HIV patients develop Eosinophilic Folliculitis has not been discovered yet, but researchers have found this folliculitis contains the same fungus with a yeast-like base as Pityrosporum Folliculitis.

Carbuncles and Boils – The cause of boils and carbuncles is bacterial staph infection in the hair follicles. Sudden and painful red or pink bumps are the signs of a boil with the skin surrounding the bumps becoming puffy and red. Within a few hours, the bump will fill with pus which causes it to grow larger and become increasingly painful. It will eventually burst and drain but could leave a scar. The smaller boils, if left alone, will heal and leave no scars. Carbuncles are similar to boils as they are simply a more densely populated group of boils and show up on the back, shoulders, thighs or neck. Because there is more infection in carbuncles than a single boil, there is more risk for scaring, plus they take longer to heal.

Types of Superficial Folliculitis

PseudofolliculitisBarbae – When the hair follicles in a man's beard area becomes inflamed, Pseudofolliculitis barbae is most likely the cause. The small shaved hairs are curving and curling back into the skin and causing the redness and inflammation; some men may also be left with keloid scars, a dark raised scar on their beard area and neck.

TineaBarbae – This folliculitis is also found in a man's beard. However, the itchy white bumps are caused by a fungus and not a bacterium like Pseudofolliculitis Barbae. When Tinea Barbae is at its worst, the white bumps are inflamed and pus-filled, then after a few days they will burst and crust over. Some men report swollen lymph nodes and fevers along with their Tinea Barbae folliculitis rash.

Staphylococcal Folliculitis – This is one of the more common superficial folliculitis skin conditions as it can appear anywhere on the body hair follicles exist. Staphylococcal folliculitis is white, itchy, pus-filled bumps. Barber's itch is what it's called when this condition occurs in a man's beard. When the bacteria Staphylococcus aureus (staph) infects hair follicles the result is Staphylococcal folliculitis. Many people do not realize that various strands of staph bacteria live on our skin all the time and do not cause us harm. But when we have a wound or cut, the staph bacteria can enter our bodies and cause problems. Different injures to the skin, such as shaving, paper cuts and simple scratching, could introduce the staph bacteria into the blood system and cause staphylococcal folliculitis.

Pityrosporum Folliculitis – This superficial folliculitis skin condition shared by teenage boys and adult men and creates lingering, itchy red pustules typically located on the chest and back and occasionally on the face, neck, upper arms and shoulders. Pityrosporum folliculitis is triggered by a yeast-like infection and can be painful in some individuals.

Pseudomonas Folliculitis – Pseudomonas folliculitis is also referred to as "Hot Tub Folliculitis" because among the areas in which the pseudomonas bacteria grows well is a hot tub. This is because the pH and chlorine levels are not regulated properly. An individual could see their first symptoms of Pseudomonas folliculitis within about eight hours to 5 days after their exposure to this bacterium. They would see a red rash area of round bumps that are extremely itchy. Later, they would become pus-filled blister-like bumps. This type of folliculitis condition will appear to be worse around the areas of your bathing suit where the contaminated waters will remain against your skin for longer periods of time.

Herpetic Folliculitis – This superficial folliculitis takes place after someone unintentionally scrapes or cuts open a cold sore while shaving. When this happens, small blister form in the hair follicles in the area directly around the cold sores vicinity. They fill with the herpes simplex virus from the cold sore and you end up with herpetic folliculitis.

Malassezia Folliculitis – This superficial folliculitis is similar to Staphylococcal folliculitis but the raised bumps are not red but yellow and pale. Malassezia folliculitis is created by a fungus introduced to the hair follicles and can leave scars.

Razor Folliculitis – This superficial folliculitis is seen a lot in women who shave different parts of their body hair. Men can also develop razor folliculitis on their necks for the same reason. When someone shaves the hair off their skin, their pores are left open and vulnerable for invasion from fungus. When you have completed shaving, the infected area will instantly start to swell. The scarring stage of razor folliculitis is called Majocchi granuloma and when the skin reaches this phase, the individual should refrain from shaving until their folliculitis is completely cleared up.

Tufted Folliculitis – Tufted folliculitis is typically found on the scalp but is unlike scalp lesions or dandruff. With Tufted folliculitis, the hairs growing in a particular area of the scalp will fall out due to too much scarring creating a bald spot where hair is unlikely to grow back.

Oil Folliculitis – Oil folliculitis is also known as "Allergic Folliculitis" because its main cause is from exposure to various chemical skincare products, deodorants, cosmetics, toothpastes and many other toiletries. Each person will react to an allergen in their own unique way, but most individuals who develop oil folliculitis will have red, inflamed rashes on or near the site of contact.

Folliculitis Barbae-the Itchy Beast Living under Your Skin

When hair follicles become clogged, infected or are otherwise unable to host a strand of hair in a healthy environment, the body shuts down the opening or follicle. Folliculitis means "the inflammation of hair follicles" and barbae is a derivative of the Latin word "barba" which means beard.

Folliculitis barbae is a skin condition occurring in men who shave and is due to a bacterial or viral infection in the hair follicles. If you cannot successfully treat or alleviate the pain and itching at home, you will need to seek medical attention for an anti-fungal or antibiotic medication.

Causes of Folliculitis Barbae

The bacteria *Staphylococcus aureus* (*S. aureus*) is typically the cause of folliculitis barbae in men who shave their beards. However, beards which are unshaven can also be infected with folliculitis barbae but it is not as common. This type of bacterial infection can spread to other parts of the face by an unclean razor, your hands or a towel. There is another way you can become infected and that is if the *Staphylococcus aureus* (*S. aureus*) is in your nose. It could be there and you would not even know it. When you blow your nose or simply breathing can bring the bacteria down to your beard and mustache.

Folliculitis barbae is typically located at the top of a hair follicle where the hair protrudes from the skin. If the infection is deep and down near the bulb of the hair follicle, than your immune system may make it more difficult to rid your body of the infection.

Symptoms of Folliculitis Barbae

The symptoms of folliculitis barbae look fairly similar to other folliculitis skin conditions. Depending on the facial skin, if you have a beard or are clean shaven, the spots may look slightly different. Most of the folliculitis barbae bumps are going to be red, swollen, and tender to the touch and with an infected yellow spot at the top.

Ingrown hairs, known as pseudofolliculitis, can look, feel and act similar to folliculitis barbae. A magnifying glass can help you clearly see ingrown hairs if you are unsure which condition you are experiencing. You may also want to seek the advice of your primary care physician or a dermatologist. The doctor will take a sample of the pus and view it under a microscope. This will help him determine which antibiotic would be the best to help remove the bacterial infection from your body. However, if your infection does not clear up within a few day, the doctor may ask you to return for a swab of the inside of your nose. This will help decide if there may be an infection you or someone else in your home has and it is simply hidden.

Treatment Options for Folliculitis Barbae

You will need to see a doctor who will most likely prescribe a 5 or 10 day course of antibiotics to clear up the underlying cause, the infection. Antibiotics come in tablet form or a topical cream which would be applied to the affected areas 1-3 times a day. You may also need an antibiotic ointment for your nostrils to stop the reinfection from nasal passages. For chronic inflammation, some doctors will prescribe an antibiotic or antiseptic steroid cream in a mild formula.

Changing Shaving Habits

Switch to an antiseptic lotion for shaving instead of a shave gel or shaving cream. However, using a shaving gel is always preferred over a cream.

Begin by reducing the chance of reinfection from contaminated razors. Take any removable metal parts off the razor and either run them through a dishwasher or place them in a pan of boiling water for 3 to 5 minutes.

Use an antiseptic solution that contains alcohol to soak and clean plastic parts of a razor. Do this after each shave to prevent any bacteria or any other germs from living on the razor until the next time you use it.

Folliculitis or Ingrown Hair – What's the Difference?

According to longstanding medical research, a single strand of hair growing out of a hair follicle is actually the result of dead cells plus the protein keratin. Hair growth is rather slow, only about ¼ inches each month and the hair is always in one of two stages: resting or active. And we never grow or create new hair follicles; those are decided before we are born by genetics.

For both teenage boys and young girls, shaving seems to simply be another exciting rite of passage into a chore adults don't like much. Once teens shave a couple hundred times, they too become disenchanted with this "normal" activity and may look for a shortcut like "dry" shaving. What they end up with is ingrown hairs and symptoms of painful, itchy bumps. These bumps are essentially a hair with a jagged or sharp edge, which has grown back down into the skin instead of up and out of the hair follicle like normal hairs. You may not notice an ingrown hair or even suffered itching at the ingrown hair sight for a few days after you shaved that area. Hairs which have been freshly shaved are somewhat "traumatized" and will need about two days to begin growing again.

The Difference between Folliculitis and Ingrown Hairs

Folliculitis is a skin condition produced by an infection of the hair follicles, typically the bacteria *Staphylococcus aureus* (*S. aureus*). The symptoms are an itchy patch of inflamed bumps, some of which are filled with a white or yellow pus.

Ingrown hairs are almost always the result of tweezing, shaving or waxing and when the regrown hair grows back into the hair follicle or under the skin.

Both folliculitis and ingrown hairs will occur anywhere on the body hair grows and can be unsightly and painful. Ingrown hairs are more prevalent among men of Hispanic origin as well as African American men. These appear in single episodes although one might have several in a single area depending on the amount of shaving, waxing or tweezing. The pus-filled blisters are painful.

Folliculitis will also have a pus-filled blister although it will almost always have a single hair growing out of the center of the blister whereas an ingrown hair will not have a hair sticking out of the center. The hair will be growing downward or under the skin. This will be the best way to tell the difference.

Types of Ingrown Hairs

There are two types of ingrown hairs: Transfollicular and Extrafollicular.

Transfollicular is when a hair never leaves or grows outside the follicle. This is because the hair has a natural curl to it and will curl back into the follicle, before growing outside the skin, and buildup fluid or pus and cause irritation.

Extrafollicular is when a hair grows out of the follicle but then reenters the skin, either directly inside the same follicle or a nearby hair follicle or pore.

Treatments

Folliculitis – Treating folliculitis may simply require patience because most of the time, this skin condition will clear up on its own. However, if you find it will not go away or it keeps coming back, you will need to see your primary care physician or a dermatologist. A doctor may prescribe a topical or oral antibiotic or an antifungal medication such as Mupirocin or Dicloxacillin.

Ingrown Hairs – Until the ingrown hair works its way out or you can successfully treat it, you will need to stop shaving, tweezing or waxing in that area. You might want to try an antibiotic cream or ointment, retinoid cream or a corticosteroid ointment to help alleviate the pain and discomfort.

If the ingrown hair has created a pustule, you will want to express it, carefully, to help promote faster healing. You can do this with a regular sewing needle which you have cleaned with rubbing alcohol. You can gently puncture the pustule and allow the pus to drain, then clean the area with a warm wash cloth. Dab a little antibiotic ointment on the ingrown hair and cover it with a bandage to help keep it clean and dry.

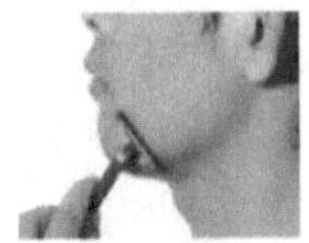

The Zen Method – Some skin experts recommend simply relaxing your muscles throughout the shaving or waxing process. Do not pull your skin when shaving and simple shave with a relaxed facial expression or relaxed leg muscle. This might help prevent folliculitis and some ingrown hairs, but these skin conditions will still happen on a regular basis.

Stimulation Method – Another option to avoid as many ingrown hairs as possible is to briskly rub your skin with a sponge specifically designed for exfoliating or a towel after each shower or bath. This could not only help all of the hairs on your body stand up, but it might also prevent the bacteria from entering the hair follicles which is the main cause of the folliculitis skin condition. You will need to be careful not to rub too harshly and avoid damaging the hair or any existing folliculitis, acne or other skin conditions.

Laser Hair Removal – Many dermatologists and skin care experts recommend laser hair removal because this procedure not only removes the hair, it removes the hair follicle, the part of the body where everything becomes infected or ingrown in the first place.

Shaving – Perhaps the easiest and best way to avoid both ingrown hairs and folliculitis of various kinds is to learn proper shaving techniques. What you may have learned when you were younger could not be the correct way and could be a major contributing factor to your recurring folliculitis or ingrown hairs.

Proper Shaving Techniques

Women

Nearly all women shave as often as men. They shave the tricky and uneven areas under their arms, the delicate bikini line and their legs pretty much on a daily basis, especially during the warmer weather months. When a woman does not shave these areas, in some cultures, she is viewed as "un-kept" or "too natural" while in other cultures the unshaved woman is seen as beautiful.

Step One – You will need to soak the area you are wanting to shave in very warm or fairly hot water. This helps the hair become more pliable and softer. Allowing your hair to soak at least 10 minutes will give you an easier time when shaving. Your hair will cut easier and not have a ragged or sharp edge which can lead to ingrown hairs.

Step Two – Slather on a good quality thick shaving gel. Always use a gel instead of a cream. Shaving gels are thicker and help keep the hairs standing up straighter than creams.

Step Three – Use a clean razor each time. If using a disposable razor, be sure to throw it away after each use. If using it more than one time, clean the blade with alcohol each time. Always use a single blade razor.

Step Four – Shave with downward strokes because this is the way your hair grows. Shaving with the hair growth instead of against it may seem a little "weird" at first, but it is the best way to prevent infection and ingrown hairs. You will also want to only pass the razor over your skin one time before rinsing it and moving on to another part of your skin.

Step Five – Sooth on a generous amount of a bump-minimizing antiseptic. These work great for reducing the number of ingrown hairs and help to keep skin soft and smooth longer.

Men

Taking the time to properly shave, from beginning to end, is one of the most significant things you can do for treating and preventing folliculitis barbae from taking over your face and your life. Most men do not have time each day to invest in their shaving routine, but for something this important, you should make time or maybe, you will need to get used to the beard look.

Step One – Using a clean wash cloth, soak it in very warm to hot water for a few moments. Then apply the wet wash cloth to the affected area for approximately 10 to 15 minutes, pressing firmly but not hard. This will help to make the skin more pliable while allowing the pus, which has built up over time, to drain.

Step Two – Apply a thin layer of oatmeal soothing lotion to your face. An oatmeal moisturizing lotion will help relieve irritation and stop further dryness. Dryness will intensify skin irritation and could cause the spread of bacteria.

Step Three – Change the blades before each shave and use a higher quality razor blade. Single blades are also better than the multi-blade razors to help prevent folliculitis and ingrown hairs. You may also want to consider switching to a superior quality electric razor. When using a regular razor, toss the razor blade after each shave or disinfect and clean it with alcohol to kill lingering bacteria. Keep several cotton balls soaking in alcohol for cleaning your electric razor to save time, toss them when done.

Step Four – To prepare your face for shaving, steam it in the shower with very warm water or with another very warm wash cloth. This should be done for roughly 10 to 15 minutes.

Step Five – Use a good quality shaving gel instead of a cream and use a generous amount for each shaving session. Never "dry" shave.

Step Six – Begin shaving, going with the growth of the hair and not against. This may seem a bit "unnatural" at first, but it will feel so much better in the end. If using a regular razor, be sure to rinse the blade after each pass over your skin. If you have a folliculitis infection, avoid shaving this area. It would be best to leave an infected space alone to completely heal before shaving that skin again.

Step Seven – Use your hands to cup water and thoroughly rinse your face. Be sure to use a clean, dry towel each day when patting your face dry, do not rub to dry.

Step Eight – Gently apply an alcohol and fragrance-free aftershave lotion. An aftershave lotion which is made of part glycolic acid will also help fight infections.

Folliculitis or Acne – What's the Difference?

For many individuals, acne and folliculitis have very similar symptoms when it appears on their skin. Both have indicators such as a cluster of red, itchy bumps with a white pus-filled head at the top. However, their causes are different and so are the treatment options.

Acne Explained

Acne is the result of a buildup of dead skin cells and oil within a hair follicle or pore. A hair follicle is attached to the sebaceous gland and when this gland produces too much sebum, a type of oil, then the pore becomes clogged and the conditions are greater for a pimple or zit to form. When the balance of sebum and dead skin cells tips too far to contain more dead skin cells than sebum and the clog or plug is closer to the skin's surface, than a blackhead if formed; if there is too much sebum and less dead skin cells then a "regular" white-head type pimple will form.

What may strike many people as odd is the fact that everyone has the bacteria *Propionibacterium acnes* on their skin normally. This bacteria uses sebum as food for growth, but during puberty it "kicks into overdrive" and individuals with more *Propionibacterium acnes* on their skin will have acne prone skin with more breakouts then other individuals. The overload of bacteria draws white blood cells to the hair follicle, which produces an enzyme. The enzyme "eats away" a portion of the wall in the follicle and this exposes it to the content of the hair follicle which quickly seeps into the surrounding skin. Through this progression, an inflammatory response is created which produces pustules or pimples, red bumps or papules and nodules. Free fatty acid bumps could also be formed which are also raised, itchy and irritating bumps.

Acne Causes

The main causes for acne include:

Stress

Poor diet

Hormones

Vitamin deficiency

Poor Diet – Although not directly connected, stress and poor diet can lead to acne through what the body produces as a result of increased stress or poor diet choices. For example, drinking too much caffeinated sugary soda and eating more chocolate because you are under additional stress does not directly produce acne on your face or anywhere on your body. However, this combination of powerful sugar and caffeine overload will have your body produce more cortisol hormone which will contribute to clogging your pores with excess sebum. Also, when we are stressed, we tend to avoid proper hygiene such as washing our face at night before going to bed. A day's worth of dirt and oil built up on the delicate skin on our face and then rubbed in while we are sleeping will also contribute to clogged pores and result in acne.

Eating a healthy diet rich in real foods such as fresh fruits, vegetables, limited lean meats and limited low-fat dairy would be ideal to help protect your skin against environmental pollutants and free radicals which can both damage the skin in a number of ways.

Stress – While it is always beneficial to reduce the stress in your life, it is not always a practical matter. What you can do is adjust your attitude towards stress, which is basically how you deal with the stress and how it is affecting your life and your health. You could start with exercise and meditation. Always start slow; there is no rush to win a marathon on one of your first outings. You can start by walking a little further each day and soon you will find you are not only feeling physically better, but you are dealing with the stresses of your daily life on a more even and calmer level. Plus, you will notice that exercise pumps more blood through your body and to your skin, which helps to flush out the bacteria and toxins and keep it healthier.

You will not be able to meditate for a long time at first, or even need to. You do not have to sit cross-legged like a Buddha to reap the benefits of meditation; you can sit or lie down, whichever is most comfortable for you. If your mind wonders, which everyone's mind does, notice it and gently guide it back to your breathing and your meditative thoughts. It might be helpful to find a CD of meditation prompts or guided narratives to help you, but it is not necessary. Studies have shown that individuals who meditate even several times a week are calmer and overall happier with their lives.

Hormones and Vitamin Deficiencies – If you believe you might have a hormone and/or vitamin deficiency, a doctor could prescribe one or both of these to bring the amounts back to the correct levels for your age, gender and weight. A daily vitamin may be helpful, but without proper testing to see which vitamins you are deficient in, you may be contributing to your acne or folliculitis skin conditions.

What Sets Your Skin Ablaze – Itchy Triggers

For each individual, there could be a number of different triggers that causes their skin to begin to itch. Folliculitis is considered a result of a bacterial infection or a yeast infection, but your hair follicles could also become damaged and clogged by other means.

Possible Triggers

There are many different things we do and don't do to our skin which can become a trigger that leads to folliculitis.

Improper Shaving – When you shave against the natural growth of the hair, the remaining portion of the hairs become jagged and sharp. Some of these hairs could grow back down into the hair follicle and cause folliculitis. Other small stubs of hair can become "catchers' mitts" for dirt and germs which could enter the hair follicle and start an infection.

Tight Clothing – When your clothing is too tight, it can rub against the tiny hairs, causing friction and irritation. When the hair follicles are red and irritated, they become swollen and can attract more bacteria to the open pores in the skin. Some of the bacteria might be the natural "good" bacteria already located on the body while some bacteria could be from other sources and not be as good for the body or skin.

Perspiration – Sweating from hard work, exercise, heat or anxiety will cause an irritation within your hair follicles. Some of the hair follicles may swell up with the sweat inside before you are able to shower. The trapped sweat in the hair follicles can cause an infection and lead to folliculitis.

Makeup – Prolonged use of makeup can be a contributing factor in folliculitis. Wearing makeup for long periods of time, more than about 6 to 8 hours, without allowing your skin to "breath" could clog the pores or hair follicles with everyday dirt. This will lead to skin irritation and folliculitis.

Antibiotics, Medicated Creams and Ointments – Prescription antibiotics taken for long periods of time can contribute to folliculitis appearing in various parts of the body. The buildup of the medication, combined with the breakdown of one's immune system is the main contribution to folliculitis. Prescription steroid-based creams and ointments used long-term could also trigger folliculitis in many patients.

Working With or Using Certain Chemicals – When your job requires you to work with chemicals such as tar, motor oils and other vehicle fluids and chemical paint strippers or other chemical toxins can cause serious damage to hair follicles as well as to the skin itself. Even if you wear protective gloves and other clothing, breathing these types of toxic chemicals can damage not only your lungs, but your hair follicles as well.

Open Wounds – Open wounds from a surgical procedure could spread fungus or bacteria to hair follicles on the skin nearby. A cut or scrap, especially ones received from something dirty or rusty, could cause bacteria to enter the hair follicle and create the perfect environment for folliculitis.

Chronic Illness – When your immune system is compromised, such as with diabetes, HIV or Sickle-cell Anemia, then you will have a more difficult time fighting off bacteria and small infections. When a few hair follicles become infected with bacteria or fungus and someone without a compromised immune system developed folliculitis, they have a greater chance of it clearing up on its own within a few days. But because of your compromised immune system, a mild folliculitis condition could quickly turn into a severe case requiring a doctor's assistance.

Swimming Pools and Hot Tubs – When you swim in public pools, hot tubs or whirlpools, or friend's pools, you risk infections that lead to folliculitis. The reason is the pH balance is not correctly calibrated and the chlorine may be too low to kill off bacteria and other germs. When you swim in water that is not properly treated, the water will soak your bathing suit as well as cling to the skin near any clothing.

Hot Tub Folliculitis – You Mean I Could Catch This?

Hot tub folliculitis is not exactly something you can "catch" from taking a dip in a hot tub or any other public pool or public water source. However, you can become infected by the bacteria *Pseudomonas aeruginosa*, which is a direct cause of folliculitis.

When a hot tub is not properly maintained and chemically treated, it means the pH is not balanced and it is becomes open to several different bacteria strains growing among the hot waters. And when you come along to take a relaxing soak or maybe go a few laps in a pool that is under chlorinated, you become "lunch" for the bacteria, so to speak. The bacteria living in the water collects on your swimsuit and you will notice, usually anywhere from a few hours to about 5 days or longer, several small red, itchy bumps on your skin, mostly where the bands of your swimsuit rested. This is because the water becomes trapped in one or more hair follicles and that is the right condition for folliculitis.

Hot tub folliculitis is sometimes referred to as Pseudomonas Folliculitis after the bacterium that causes the infection. After the red bumps first appear, they will either go away almost as quickly or they will become darker and fill with pus. At this point the hot tub folliculitis infection should have run its course and fade away in a few short days. If the pus-filled bumps do not drain and heal on their own, and you experience fever and exhaustion, then it may be time to contact your doctor.

If your hot tub folliculitis requires treatment, your doctor will want to examine the infection first. Then the doctor will probably prescribe an oral antibiotic such as Levofloxacin or Ciprofloxacin. The doctor might combine the oral antibiotic with a topical antibiotic to make sure the infection completely heals. You may also receive an anti-itch medication to help the bumps heal without the fear of scratching them open again.

To prevent hot tub folliculitis from reoccurring, you will need to be extremely careful and attentive to where you do your hot tubing and swimming. Ask to see a maintenance record if you are going to use the water facilities at your apartment or gym. These documents will tell you if the pH and chlorine levels have been maintained and over how long. If you are visiting a friend's pool or hot tub, be sure to shower with an antibacterial soap immediately upon exiting the water and dry off with a clean towel. This will be your best defense against hot tub folliculitis.

Do You Recognize These Symptoms?

The symptoms of folliculitis vary depending on which version of the disease you are suffering from. In general, all types of folliculitis begin as an itchy, red rash of small, pin-size bumps which are the inflamed hair follicles. Here are the most common symptoms no matter which type of folliculitis you are diagnosed with.

Erythema – This is the redness and inflammation of the skin before any other symptoms appears. The skin changes colors and swells slightly, but not enough for a bump, before pus accumulates in the hair follicle.

Rashes – Red, itchy, patchy rashes are among the most common folliculitis symptoms. A rash is often the second symptom you experience that might lead you to believe you are about to suffer a folliculitis skin condition. One of the worst things you can do is starch the itchy rash. When you scratch the pus-filled bumps, you first burst open the bumps and then risk spreading the fungus or bacteria that started the rash to other parts of your skin.

Pain – This indicator of folliculitis may occur at the same time as the first two symptoms or not until later, but pain happens because the fungus or bacteria is basically "eating" its way through the hair follicles and your body is trying to stop this process and shut it down before it can do major damage. The pain may continue for a day or two after the hair follicle closes up and your body enters "repair mode".

Edema – This is a condition of the skin, which shows itself as a buildup of fluid directly under the skin's surface. The fluid produces small but noticeable bags-type bumps under the skin. Then within about a day, the pus or concentrated infection begins to form and the swelling creates a larger bump or bag.

Exhaustion and Fever – When folliculitis does not heal on its own and goes untreated, the main causes of fungus or bacteria can enter the bloodstream through the hair follicle infection. You will then need immediate medical treatment because you now have a systemic infection on your hands instead of a mild skin infection.

I Have Folliculitis *Where*?

Many individuals can't imagine where they would come in contact with infectious bacteria or fungus that could lead them to develop painful folliculitis. But what most people don't realize and are surprised to discover is that everyone, even the cleanest person on the planet, has bacteria living on their skin as well as inside their body. Furthermore, without that bacterium, their immune system would not be able to survive and they would parish.

Folliculitis is an infected hair follicle, so anywhere you have hair growing you can become infected and suffer from red, itchy, embarrassing and painful folliculitis. Scalp folliculitis occurs because the follicles on the scalp have become infected and individuals will experience folliculitis on the fine, thin hairs on their arms as well as the harder, coarse hairs on their legs. And, it should be no surprise that the red, itchy and painful pus-filled bumps can appear on their buttocks as well as in their pubic area.

How Did Folliculitis Get *There?*

There are basically two ways to get folliculitis in the pubic area:

Friction – This is typically caused by clothing rubbing the hairs this way and that and then the damaged hairs cause the follicles to become infected.

Shaving – This is the more common of the two reasons for folliculitis in the pubic area. Folliculitis from shaving is also known as barber's itch or razor burn.

Possible Treatment Options

At home, there are only a few treatment options you could try to help alleviate the pain, swell and itching.

Warm/Hot Compresses – The first option is to apply a warm to hot compress over the folliculitis pus-filled bumps. You can use a clean wash cloth or other clean cloth such as a sterile piece of gauze. Do not press hard but apply the hot cloth firmly to the infected area so the pus will drain away, taking off the pressure which is the main cause of the pain.

You can soak a clean cloth in an over-the-counter solution such as Burow's to help drain the pustule. Or, make a warm or hot compress at home using 1 tablespoon white vinegar and 1.33 cups of warm or hot water. Either of these solutions will help to draw the pus out and shrink the swelling a bit.

Antibiotic Ointment – There are several low-grade brands you could purchase over-the-counter but their strength is not very strong. You may need to contact your doctor or dermatologist for something stronger if the infection is too painful and lasts for several days.

Antibiotic Medication – A prescription for antibiotic medication would need to come from your physician or dermatologist if the folliculitis in your pubic area is persistent and painful. However, seeking medical advice would be worth the trouble in this case because folliculitis in the pubic area response quite well to antibiotics.

Prevention

There are a couple preventative measures both men and women can take to help lessen the likelihood they will develop painful folliculitis in their pubic area. These precautionary tasks are not a guarantee against developing folliculitis, but they will help a great deal towards unnecessary infections.

Wear Lose-fitting Clothing – For both men and women, their underwear does not need to be skin tight. Clothing that is too tight holds in sweat, moisture and any type of bacteria which can all lead to folliculitis. The same goes for "skinny jeans". If you feel you must wear tighter clothes, do so on an irregular basis.

Change Clothing and Sheets – If you have an infected pubic area, be sure to change your clothing often and do not wear those clothes again without washing them first. You will need to change and wash your sheets every couple days as well, even if you sleep in night clothes, the infection and other body oils can seep through your clothing and remain on the sheets for days, possibly causing a reinfection of your skin.

Proper Pubic Hair Shaving

Many men and women enjoy a clean shaven pubic area, which is perfectly fine but it can often lead to folliculitis. Proper pubic hair shaving should always be practiced to help cut down on the number of infected hair follicles in that most delicate and private area of the body. Here are several tips to follow to help you achieve a smooth, clean pubic area shave.

Choosing the Right Products

Shaving Gels and Creams – It is best to use the mildest type of shaving gel or cream available. Choose one without perfumes, dyes or other type of harsh chemicals. A product that is all natural and specifically made for delicate skin would be preferred for this gentle area and a shaving gel is also a better performer than a shaving cream.

New Razors – Do not use a cheap disposable razor or a double razor blade. Purchase a new, good quality razor for your pubic area and plan to use it only once or twice and then throw it away. You might try a razor with a "soap strip" or "lotion strip" that helps soften the hairs before they are cut by the razor. Never use an electric razor on your pubic area.

Small Sharp Scissors – It is a good idea to trim the pubic hairs before shaving that area. This allows for a closer shave as well as helping to cut down on the number of hair follicles which could become infected from ingrown hairs.

Mild Baby Oil and Aloe Vera Cream – You can use baby oil when you are done shaving to prevent pimples from forming. This should be helpful although a handful of people do experience a rash or other type of skin irritation from baby oil. If this is the case for you, use the aloe vera cream, which is used as a calming cream for inflammation.

Tweezers and Hair Conditioner – The tweezers and hair conditioner are optional items but can be helpful when it comes to removing pubic hairs. Using a good quality hair conditioner to wash your pubic hair and help them become softer if they are extremely coarse. This could take several washings with the conditioner before you see a marked difference, but it will be there.

The tweezers can be used to get the hairs in the folds and hard to reach places that a razor shouldn't go.

Shaving Your Pubic Area

Step One – Begin by carefully cutting as much of your pubic hair as you can with the sharp scissors. This will help the shaving and lessen the skin irritation and possible infection.

Step Two – To help make the hairs softer and easier to shave, soak in a hot bath or take a hot shower for 3 to 5 minutes. If you plan to use hair conditioner on your pubic hairs, this should be done the day before you plan to shave. This way the conditioner will not be fresh on the hairs or irritating the skin.

Step Three – Dry off with a clean towel and in order to allow your skin to recover from the water, wait about three minutes before beginning to shave.

Step Four – Apply the shaving gel. Do not apply too thick or too thin, you will figure out the right amount after the first time. You can always apply more or take off too much.

Step Five – Using your free hand, pull the skin taut and begin shaving in an upwards direction. The pubic hairs always grow downward and it is best to shave against the growth pattern. However, if you are susceptible to ingrown hairs, it would be better to shave with the growth pattern.

Step Six – When you've completely shaved the area, rinse several times with warm water or jump back in the shower to ensure you rinse all the shaving gel off to avoid irritation and itching. When you are sure there is no more shaving gel, pat dry with a clean towel.

Step Seven – Apply a thin layer of baby oil to prevent pimples. You can also apply the aloe vera cream to soothe and calm irritated skin.

Important Considerations

Do not shave when you first wake up in the morning or after a nap. When we are sleeping, many of the body's fluids collect under the skin. This makes skin puffier which can increase the risk of cuts and infections when shaving. Waiting 30 minutes or longer will allow the skin to relax and distribute the fluids and the hairs to extend straighter.

When looking for an aloe vera cream, do not use one with sunscreens, anti-aging properties or other types of additives you won't need and could cause skin irritation, itching and possibly an infection. Look for sensitive skin moisturizers which will be mild on this area as well as others.

If you use baby oil, do not have sex using a condom unless you take a bath or shower first to remove all traces of the baby oil. Baby oil destroys latex which most condoms are made of or have a large portion of, therefore it is recommended to shower off the oil or avoid sex until you can wash it away.

Multiple Choice Answers – The Many Cures

There are several types of medications, alternative remedies and diet changes which allow an individual with folliculitis `to control their symptoms and avoid further skin damage.

Here is a list of just a few of the many cure options:

Medication sub-categories:

Topical (applied to the skin)

Oral (pill form)

Medications are typically antibiotic or antifungal to address the infections that cause the folliculitis to appear and irritate the skin. Prescription strength antibiotic ointments which contain neomycin or mupirocin could be used to combat infectious folliculitis. If this does not work, a doctor might switch to an oral medication in a penicillinase-resistant penicillin.

Alternative Treatments

Essential Oils – Many are applied directly to the infection while others are used as a vapor and breathed to work from the inside out.

Herbal Treatments – Herbal treatments can be applied directly to a folliculitis skin infection or used as a tea and drank to benefit from the healing properties in many of the different herbs.

Acupuncture – Many believe this ancient Asian medical treatment helps to draw the heat away from the infection, helping the individual feel better.

Yoga – Practicing yoga is not necessarily a cure or treatment for folliculitis, however, this form of gentle movement and exercise encourages relaxation and encourages a better immune system which is what is needed to fight infections.

Laser Hair Treatments – Many adults will seek a professional laser hair removal treatment from a qualified technician. This type of folliculitis treatment will be permanent but should be conducted as more of a preventative measure rather than a treatment. Laser hair removal destroys the hair and much of the follicle the hair grows from which in turns helps to prevent folliculitis from forming.

Severe Cases

When you have a severe case of folliculitis, which does not heal on its own with a home remedy or prescription medications, your doctor may recommend a small procedure to drain the pustule. You should never try to "pop" or otherwise "remove" a folliculitis infection yourself because of the risk of spreading the infection to other nearby hair follicles.

I Thought I Knew How to Wash My Skin

Proper skin hygiene is extremely important for every one of all ages and for both men and women. There is some research that points to an increased amount of folliculitis appearing in teenagers and young adults, but this skin infection can affect anyone at any age. The best defense is to properly care for your skin at all times, every day and to adjust your routine only to accommodate the changing of the seasons.

Why Maintain Proper Skin Hygiene

You need to remove dirt, microbes and dead skin cells from your skin's surface daily to avoid clogging the pores which can cause folliculitis and other skin issues. At the same time, it is vital to preserve the natural oils and fats, known as extracellular lipids on the skin's outer layer, known as the stratum corneum.

What Skin Needs

Your skin needs both lipids and moisture to sustain its protective barrier, the outer layer. Your skin also needs a healthy dose of what's known as "resident" microbes. These are microbes or organisms that live on your body but do you no harm. They actually help protect you from the harmful attacks of pathogens that do cause diseases. When you clean your skin too much, you strip away the resident microbes and leave your skin susceptible to infection.

To help your skin from the inside, eat a well-balanced healthy diet that promotes glowing, strong skin. You will also want to reduce damage from environmental factors such as the sun, smog and other chemical toxins.

How-to Clean Your Skin

To remove daily grease and dirt, choose a skin cleaner or mild soap that contain emollients and moisturizers. Be sure the soap or skin cleaner you use is not overly alkaline or acidic and has mild-surface active ingredients to avoid stripping the "good" bacteria from your skin. Soaps with detergents and harsh chemicals will do the same.

Using too much antibacterial soap or skin cleaner containing antibacterial chemicals can strip away your skin's oils, fats and protective layers. Save this type of soap for hand washing, but use it sparingly here as well. When washing your hands, do not scrub hard although you should gently rub your hands together for at least 15-20 seconds with the soap to insure they are clean. Many germ-avoiding safety sites recommend singing the *Alphabet Song* while rubbing your hands together to provide the proper amount of time for the soap to clean your hands.

Always use lukewarm or warm water when bathing, showering or washing your hands. Never use hot or very hot water because it will wash away the resident microbes and could burn your skin.

Each time you use soap or a skin cleaner, be sure to rinse well with warm water. You do not want to leave any type of cleaner on your skin because it could cause drying as well as become itching or lead to an infection.

Dry your skin with a fresh, clean towel each time and always use a patting motion, never rub with the towel. Rubbing causes friction that can break and otherwise damage hair which can lead to folliculitis.

Always select products for sensitive skin with no dyes, perfumes or harsh chemicals; even if your skin is not particularly sensitive, it will be if you don't take care of it.

Wash your face before you go to bed, no matter how tired you are or where you are, just do it. If you can, wash and pat dry your face and apply moisturizer and medications about an hour before turning in to bed. This will allow them to be fully absorbed before rubbing on the pillow.

Change your sheets twice a week and your pillowcase more often. Dirt, oil, grease and even infections can get trapped in the sheets and pillowcases and then transfer back on your skin. If you have folliculitis or any other skin infection, change the sheets and pillowcase daily, washing them before putting them back on the bed.

Unless your hands are clean, do not touch your face. Your face has a slightly more delicate skin surface and bacteria "feeds" folliculitis as well as acne.

Choose a non-comedogenic or non-occlusive make-up to reduce pore-clogging that could lead to folliculitis or acne. Remember, all make-up can clog pores so use as little as possible for the shortest period of time needed, then gently clean your face.

Clean or replace make-up sponges and brushes often and if you have folliculitis or another skin infection, throw out all make-up and applicators so as not to re-infect yourself.

Stop Feeding Your Folliculitis-Proper Diet for Great Skin

Currently, there is no direct evidence which forms a connection from what we eat and the development of folliculitis; however, there are many foods we consume which can contribute to weakening the immune system and deteriorating our overall health. When our bodies are not healthy, they can develop diseases and are more susceptible to infections.

Here is a list of diet and food "dos" and "don'ts" to help you become healthier and keep bacteria, which can cause folliculitis, at bay.

Omega-3 Fatty Acids – Eat more foods rich in Omega-3 fatty acids such as wild Alaskan salmon, fortified eggs, walnuts, sardines and flax seeds. The reason the body needs Omega-3 fatty acid is for cell health. This particular fatty acid helps create a stronger cell wall which allows water to remain within the cell. When this happens, skin cells look plumper, more vibrant and healthier.

Whole Grains – Eat more whole grains such as oats and whole wheat products because they have shown to possess anti-inflammatory properties and are full of antioxidants.

Blueberries – Eat more blueberries because they are rich in antioxidants and help fight against free radicals which cause DNA damage and skin cell damage from UV radiation and pollution.

Almonds – Almonds are rich in monounsaturated fat and filled with vitamin E. Eating a handful (half a cup) of almonds a few times a week will help your skin look younger by keeping the cell membranes intact and strong.

Spinach – Eating more of this green, dark leafy food helps put a super-charged antioxidant in your body where it will slow down skin cancer cells and repair other skin cells damaged by the sun. Spinach contains potassium, folate, lutein and fiber; all which can help restore cells and repair DNA.

Water – Good, clean water is extremely important to maintain a healthy body and glowing skin. Drink filtered or purified water as much as possible throughout the day. Water helps to flush the toxins out of the body through urination and sweating and the purified or filtered water works best to prevent adding the toxins back into the body or getting them caught in the pours during elimination such as sweating.

What *Not to Do* to Have Healthier Skin

High Carbs – Eating large quantities of high carb foods such as cookies, sugar, white flour products like bread and junk food should be avoided. All of these types of foods, the ones with mostly "empty calories", can contribute to clogging your attires. Plus, large amounts of sugar and grease can lead to increased stress and anxiety which leads to increased perspiration which leads to folliculitis.

Dairy Intake – When you consume too much high fat dairy such as cheese, full-fat yogurt and ice cream, you risk contributing to acne and other pore-clogging disease. Aim for eating fat-free or low-fat varieties of dairy on a limited basis during the week to prevent sugar spikes and clogging your pores.

Salt Intake – Decrease your salt intake as much as possible not only for the treatment and prevention of folliculitis, but for your overall better health. Tissue swelling is the result of too much sodium and when your skin is swelled, hair follicles become restricted and can become infected easier. Try to eat fresh vegetables instead of the can varieties. If you do use can vegetables, check the sodium levels and rinse the contents to help remove a little sodium.

Candy – Avoid all candies because they are loaded with sugar and will dull your skin as well as cause wrinkles. Too much sugar harms the elastin and collagen which is the critical fibers which hold your skin firm and keep it youthful. The sugar will cause your skin to become dry and can also cause sagging in some spots.

Traditional Medicines for Folliculitis

There are several traditional medications doctors will prescribe for treating folliculitis on the skin. Some of them are topical which should be applied directly to the affected area while other medications are in pill form and work from the inside out. Many doctors will advise their patients to us both oral and topical medications to speed up the treatment time of folliculitis.

Here is a list of some of the most common medications for treating folliculitis infections. However, each doctor is unique in his or her methods and not every doctor has access to all research done on folliculitis and the medications that work or those that do not work.

Oral Medications

Dapsone (Aczone)

Ciprofloxacin (Cipro)

Famciclovir (Famvir)

Linezolid (Zyvox)

Dicloxacillin

Mupirocin (Bactroban, Centany)

Acyclovir (Zovirax)

Rifampin (Rifadin)

Cephalexin (Keflex)

Valacyclovir (Valtrex)

Minocycline (Minocin, Dynacin, Solodyn)

Topical Medications

Topical Antibiotics

Clindamycin (Cleocin, Cleocin T, ClindaMax, Clindagel, Evocin)

Erythromycin (Akne-mycin, Ery)

Topical Antifungal

Econazole (Spectazole)

Ciclopirox (Loprox)

Ketoconazole (Nizole, Xolegel, Extina)

Corticosteroids

Halobetasol (Ultravate) – Topical

Triamcinolone (Kenalog-10, Kenalog-40, Aristospan) – Topical or injection

Clobetasol propionate (Temovate, Clobex, Cormax) – Topical creams, gels, ointments, foams or lotions

Flucinonide (Vanos) – Topical creams and ointments

30-Days to Relief With Natural Treatment Options

Many individuals believe in alternative medicine and their treatments to work best for relieving their skin of folliculitis. There are several different options when it comes to treatments deemed alternative or what your doctor may not consider writing a prescription for. Some of them may not work for you while others will help clear up the painful red itching skin in a matter of days. As will all medical type treatments use caution and if your symptoms worsen or if you become ill, seek medical assistance immediately.

Essential Oils

Using essential oils as either a topical application or as a vapor to be breathed in for a limited time could help reduce many of the symptoms of folliculitis. Some "full strength" essential oils should be avoided due to the dangers of burning or further infection. Always read warning labels carefully before applying.

Tea Tree Oil – This essential oil has both an antifungal and antibacterial in potent quantities that when applied to the affected folliculitis area will attack the infection and clear it up in a matter of days in most individuals.

Oil of Lemon – Either the essential oil or the oil used as a vaporized treatment has been shown to destroy strains of staphylococcus and many other bacteria strains.

Lavender Oil – Folliculitis is caused by bacteria, Staphylococcus S aureus the most common but also Enterobacter, Proteus, Klebsiella or Pseudomonas could be the cause. Oil of Lavender has antibacterial properties and has been shown to fight against many of these bacteria.

Oregano Oil – This is antibacterial and antifungal oil that can be used topically. This essential oil also has anti-inflammatory, anti-parasitic and anti-oxidant properties which help your skin look and feel its best.

Rose Oil – This essential oil is a bactericide and at the same time inhibits the growth of bacteria. It will soothe inflammation as well as help with healing scars.

Rosemary Oil – This is an anti-inflammatory and antibacterial essential oil that helps to treat all types of skin disorders.

Thyme Oil – This is an essential oil which kills bacteria, helps to protect wounds from becoming diseased or further infected and heals after marks or scars.

Bergamot Oil – This type of essential oil comes in several varieties and the citric type is best because of its antibiotic properties as well as its ability to heal cuts and scars as well as suppress pain.

Other Alternative Treatment Options

Yoga – The practice of yoga may not be a direct treatment for folliculitis, but this ancient type of stretching and movement will help to remove toxic buildup within the body and promote a healthier immune system, everything that is needed to ward off infections that lead to folliculitis.

Meditation – Like yoga, it is not a direct treatment for folliculitis but when your mind is calmer and clearer, you will not only feel better, but you will be able to take better care of yourself. You will find you engage in more of the recommendations that help treat and prevent folliculitis then you did before you began meditating. For example, you might start washing your face before jumping into bed every night and drinking more water where before, you did not do these helpful things.

Acupuncture – Acupuncture has been shown to help relieve the pain and inflammation of folliculitis in some individuals by drawing the heat away from the infected follicles. If you are going this route, be sure to use a certified acupuncturist. They will not only know where to insert the needles, they will use disposable ones to keep you from further infection and harm.

Home Remedies and Natural Cures

There are many home remedies and natural cures for folliculitis you may try, but as with traditional medication and alternative treatments, not everything works for everyone. And always use caution. Just because something is labeled natural does not mean there might not be side effects. Although not as common, you could be allergic to or have a reaction to an all-natural ingredient.

Vinegar – White or apple cider vinegar, both diluted can be used to create an acidic environment for the bacteria that causes the folliculitis infections. Studies show that bacteria cannot survive in acidic solutions and this is why vinegar works well as a natural treatment. Apply sparingly as it will temporarily burn or sting the skin.

Blackstrap Molasses – Blackstrap molasses is basically what's left after the final extraction of sugar from raw sugar cane or after the third boiling. This is considered a "super food" containing several vitamins, minerals and iron. The overall benefits to your body can help not only treat folliculitis but treat acne and other skin conditions. Mix 1 teaspoon with hot water, milk, soymilk, tea or many other beverages at least once a day for best results.

Fatty Acids – Increasing your intake of Omega-3 fatty acids in your diet is good but the Omega-6 fatty acids cannot be consumed through your diet in large enough quantities to make a difference, they need to be taken in pill form. Omega-6 fatty acids supplements are the GLA (gamma-linolenic acid) which is needed for healthy nails, hair and skin. Some of the best dietary supplements to try are borage oil, evening primrose oil and black currant oil. Fish oil supplements are also a good choice.

Cleavers – This herb supports the lymphatic system and helps to cure staph infections and abscesses while reducing the swelling of the lymph nodes.

Echinacea – This herb has antibiotic properties and can be taken in pill form to help treat folliculitis.

Turmeric Powder – This herb is part of the ginger family and has anti-inflammatory properties. Mix 1 teaspoon of the bright yellow powder with a small amount of water and swallow up to 4 times a day.

Goldenseal – There are two ways to use this versatile herb, internally and as a topical treatment. When your symptoms first appear, Goldenseal should be taken in pill form to help lessen the infection. You can also use the powder form of Goldenseal root as a paste when mixed with a small amount of water. Dab a small amount of the past on the affected skin two to three times a day.

Garlic – This herb has antibacterial properties and can be consumed as a food additive (3 gloves a day) or 3 capsules per day. Some individuals have had limited results with a garlic paste but there is a burning sensation as well as the lingering odor.

Allopathic Treatments for Folliculitis

A dermatologist is an allopathic physician. An allopathic doctor is a doctor who uses pharmaceutical medications, scientific tests and surgery to diagnose and treat their patients and will not consider alternative treatment options.

Allopathic Doctors May Use:

X-rays and other radiological-based diagnostic tools

Blood tests

Physical examinations

Skin scraping for lab culture diagnostic testing

Antibiotic and antifungal topical medications

Antibiotic and antifungal oral medications

Severe or Recurrent Folliculitis Treatment

For recurring or severe folliculitis, which is likely caused by staphylococcal bacteria, your doctor will probably prescribe a 7 or 10 day course of antibiotics like penicillin. Prescriptions for newer medications such as Fluoroquinolones or Vancomycin are on the rise because the recent strands of staph infections have become stronger and more resistant to penicillin and other common "go-to" antibiotics.

Intravenous – Intravenous antibiotics will be delivered to those individuals with the most serious infections. This type of antibiotic delivery system could last for up to six weeks and used to kill staph infections in and around the eye as well as other places on the face.

Surgery – A small percentage of individuals with serious infections end up needing surgery to drain an abscess or even remove them from internal organs, implanted devices or shunts. The majority of individuals who contract staph infections will recover after a short period of time, especially if they are healthy before they become sick. People with slightly weakened immune systems or other health issues may have a harder time recovering from a staph infection but it is possible.

Are Laser Treatments the Right Choice for Your Folliculitis?

When an individual has persistent or severe folliculitis, they may want to consider laser hair removal as one of their treatment options; however, this type of treatment could be right for some and wrong for others. In some individuals, this treatment could be more of a reinforcement or aggravator of their condition. And for others, laser hair treatments will cause an area of folliculitis to appear where there was none but it should be a temporary issue.

How Laser Hair Removal Works to Treat Folliculitis

A certified laser hair removal specialist or technician will prepare your skin and then position the laser over the affected area. When the laser is turned on, usually for only a few seconds per hair to be removed, a bright and intense light is sent down the shaft of hair and into the root below the skins surface. This is where the energy from the laser turns into heat and the root of the hair absorbs the heat. The absorbed heat is what destroys the root or bulb of the hair so that it will no longer grow. The dead hair will either dissolve or be expelled from the follicle and should not grow back. Sometimes the laser's intense heat and energy is not absorbed fully by the entire root and the hair grows back. In that case, multiple treatments may be required to be successful.

What Happens During a Laser Hair Removal Treatment Session

When it comes to laser hair removal treatments, the biggest fear for the majority of individuals is pain. Although different lasers produce varying degrees of a slight burning sensation and every individual has a different level of pain tolerance, the pain is minor and temporary. Some spas and doctor's offices offer a topical anesthetic to mildly numb or dull the skin in preparation for the laser. There are also several "cooling systems" on the market that you might inquire about when making your appointment. These are also designed to help reduce discomfort and pain.

Laser Hair Removal Aftercare

Your doctor or laser hair removal technician should give you specific instructions about caring for your recently treated skin. However, care should be taken when it comes to increased redness or swelling. These are temporary symptoms, but if they do not disappear within a day or two, you will need to contact the clinic where your procedure was performed.

Many who perform laser hair removal recommend exfoliating the day after receiving your treatment to help circulation and remove dead hair and dead skin cells. This is a critical step because dead hairs and dead skin cells can reenter the hair follicles, become infected and cause folliculitis. Another important step is to moisturize. This is to help ensure the treatment area stays soft and not dry out.

When Laser Hair Removal Causes Folliculitis

Because your skin is a delicate organ and some areas are more sensitive than others, you may experience the development of folliculitis rather than the cure or elimination of the painful bumps and pustules. Folliculitis as a result of laser hair removal should not be bacterial or fungal in nature, especially if you have chosen a qualified laser hair removal specialist or doctor. If the folliculitis from your treatment does not disappear after two days, notify the office where you received your treatment. This could mean you have an infection due to some lack of cleanliness during your procedure or you could have deep folliculitis in which you will need to see a dermatologist for other treatment options.

Food Allergens and Folliculitis

The bulk of individuals who think they have food allergies are confusing food intolerances with food allergies. A food allergy can send someone to the hospital and if their condition is not treated immediately, it could lead to so much swelling that forms a lack of oxygen and even death. Food intolerances cause irritation and an uncomfortable feeling in the stomach and intestines that typically dissipate after the food has finished processing its way through the body.

Common Foods Which Cause Allergies

Across the board, researchers have found that the same foods seem to cause the majority of allergies in people.

Nuts – Peanuts, Brazilian nuts, hazelnuts, walnuts, almonds, cashews and pecans

Seafood – Lobster, crab, oysters, shrimp and fish

Other Foods – Cow's milk, eggs, wheat, corn and citrus fruits

When you consume a food you are allergic to, your body will rebel against it by sending out histamines to fight the harmful substance it feels is "invading" it.

If you suffer from eczema, certain foods and food allergies can intensify the itching, and aggregate the red, dry patches. Other foods have also been linked to increase acne in those who already are prone to suffer from this frustrating and often embarrassing skin condition. However, there is no scientific evidence that food allergies cause folliculitis.

The Food – Fungal Infection Connection

If your doctor confirms your folliculitis is caused by a fungal infection, then there could be a connection between the foods you consume and your folliculitis. Eating too many refined carbohydrates, foods with lots of sugar as well as yeast and moldy foods can lead to an overgrowth of yeast in the body. And too much yeast causes fungal infections which are often the cause of folliculitis.

Sugar and refined carbs are the fuel the yeast needs to grow and when you eat too much, your body produces an overgrowth of yeast, mainly in your intestines, but in women yeast can grow to excessive proportions in the vaginal area as well. Also, what happens when yeast is fed too much sugar, it produces ethanol alcohol and acetaldehyde, a more toxic form of alcohol as the yeast ferments in the body.

Foods That Contribute to Yeast Overgrowth

Sugar – Foods that contain sugar should be restricted or eliminated. They include foods that contain honey, glucose, fructose, maltose, sorbitoal, lactose, mannitol, molasses and maple syrup

Processed and Packaged Foods – Foods which have been pre-packaged or processed such as boxed, bottled or canned items, often contain excess sugar and salt

Pre-packaged foods include – microwavable and ready-to-eat meals, donuts, packaged cookies, packaged bakery cakes, candy, frozen foods and breakfast cereals

Alcohol – Whiskey, beer, wine, rum, gin and brandy contain excessive amounts of sugar as well as yeast in some cases

Fungus Fit for Human Consumption– Truffles and mushrooms

Condiments – Anything pickled, marinated or fermented and anything containing mayonnaise would be filled with yeast. Others to avoid would be relishes, sauces and creams made with vinegar and mustard and soy sauce

Smoked or Processed Meets – Hot dogs, lunch meats, bacon, pastrami, corn beef, sausage, ham, canned meats and smoked fish

Milk and Cheeses – Buttermilk, sour milk products, yogurts, sour cream and moldy cheeses

Canned Foods – Sauces, soups, beans and some vegetables and fruits

Bottled Drinks – Sports drinks, artificial fruit juices, smoothies and coffees

Malted Foods – Malted milk, malted beer, candy and cereals

Dried Fruits – Figs, raisins, dates, cranberries, prunes, etc.

When you eliminate yeast from your diet and your body, you are helping to reduce the risk of yeast-related folliculitis, which can be just as painful and embarrassing as the other types.

Scalp Folliculitis

As with all types of folliculitis, it can appear anywhere you have hair growing, but folliculitis can be especially irritating and painful when it develops on the scalp. This is because your hair grows in rather dense on your scalp and the follicles may be a bit closer together there as well.

Possible Causes

Broken Hair – This could be a result of wearing hats, headbands, barrettes, ponytail bands or combing or brushing your hair too much or when it's wet.

Excessive Oil – Many individuals suffer from overactive sebum glands on their scalp. These are the glands that produce oils the body needs but in excess, and the oil will then clog the pores or hair follicles causing folliculitis.

Shaving – Men who shave their heads often suffer from scalp folliculitis just as they do when they shave their beards. The jagged, broken pieces of hair could irritate, grow back into the follicle or become infected like beard hairs.

Sweating – When you exercise or your job causes you to sweat or you perspire on your scalp for any reason, the sweat and dirt the "water droplets" collect on the way to pooling in the follicles can clog these pores and can become infected causing folliculitis.

Acne – As with skin on other parts of your body, it can often be confused with acne. A doctor can determine if your itchy, red, pus-filled bumps on your scalp are folliculitis or acne.

Home Treatment Options

There are several options you may want to try for treating your scalp folliculitis at home before seeking medical assistance from your doctor.

Warm/Hot Compress – Sometimes your scalp folliculitis needs to be drained, but do not pop the pustules or scratch them, even though they are itchy and bothersome. Use a medicated anti-itch cream for when you are going out in public or an ointment when you are home or going to bed. If your scalp folliculitis is bad, you could end up scratching, picking or popping them in your sleep. Soak a clean wash cloth in warm or hot water and a small amount of vinegar for about 3 minutes. Press the compress onto the affected folliculitis area firmly but not too hard for about 5 to 10 minutes or until the wash cloth turns cold. Do this several times a day to relieve the pressure and drain the pus and infection.

Salicylic Acid – Salicylic acid is recommended for a variety of skin conditions including folliculitis, keratosis pilaris, acne and many other skin issues. Salicylic acid is taken from willow-bark as a Beta Hydroxy Acid and will intensify the regeneration of cells. When this happens, your skin will experience less blocked follicles, which are the main cause of folliculitis, and you will experience a faster rate of skin renewal as well.

Salicylic acid, a much milder and gentler antibiotic treatment then Alpha Hydroxy Acids, acts as a drying agent when applied to the affected area with a cotton ball or other small application system. This method will reduce white-heads, exfoliate flaky, dry skin and your scalp will remain clear without buildup and breakouts far longer than other treatment procedures.

Doctor Recommended Treatment Options

When you have tried several treatment options at home and they have not given you significant relieve of your scalp folliculitis, it is time to talk to your doctor. He or she will recommend several possibilities to help alleviate the painful itching, burning and rid your scalp of the bacteria or fungus which is no doubt the root cause of your scalp folliculitis.

Your doctor might prescribe something like a mild steroid cream or lotion, which is topical, for the inflammation, as well as topical antibiotics. The antibiotics for the skin typically offered are Fusidic acid gel, clindamycin solution and erythromycin solution. The last item your doctor will prescribe is an oral antihistamine to help reduce the entire itchy infected red dry mess on your scalp.

Note of Warning

The use of Benzoyl Peroxide is similar to hydrogen peroxide when used on your hair and scalp, it is extremely damaging. Hydrogen peroxide bleaches out hair color and weakens hair down to the roots which can contribute to folliculitis. Benzoyl Peroxide may be good as an acne treatment for some people but it should never be used on your scalp.

Moisturizing Hair Mask

If you are using an antibacterial or anti-fungal shampoo several times a week, you are going to dry out your scalp and hair. You will also be depleting the much-needed vitamins and micro-nutrients your hair needs to stay vibrant and healthy. To combat this, use a home-made natural hair mask once a week to deep-condition and nourish your hair.

The reason this all-natural moisturizing hair mask works so well is due to the combination of acidity, essential vitamins, fatty acids and amino acids that combine together to replenish lost nutrients and reduce the sebum levels on the scalp.

Natural Moisturizing Hair Mask Recipe

2 egg yolks

1 cup fresh squeezed tomato juice

2 tablespoons all natural honey

1.5 cups coconut milk (be sure it is coconut milk and not coconut water)

Mix all ingredients together to form a thick paste.

Approximately one hour before washing your hair, apply the paste to your hair and scalp.

Gently massage the paste into your scalp and ends of your hair and then go about your business. You may want to put a towel around your shoulders in case of drips.

When it is time to wash your hair, rinse your hair and scalp several times with warm water to be sure the entire natural moisturizing hair mask is removed. Then continue to wash your hair as normal.

Severe Cases

If left untreated, scalp folliculitis could lead to periflolliculitis capitis or acne necrotica miliaris and need additional treatment from your doctor. If your attempt to treat your scalp folliculitis do not clear up the infection or it worsens, you will need to seek medical attention before you suffer permanent hair loss.

Preventing Folliculitis

There are many ways to prevent folliculitis from taking over your life. Prevention is not hard but it takes some planning and some patience if you already have a folliculitis infection. Here are several general tips for keeping folliculitis way from your skin.

Wash Your Hands Often – When you have an infection of folliculitis, be sure to wash your hands often with warm water and antibacterial soap. Not too often or you will strip away the "good" bacteria, but be sure to wash your hands after touching the infected area and before and after any treatment applications. Washing your hands will prevent the infection from spreading to other parts of your body or other persons you come in contact with.

Choose Showering Over Bathing – Showers are actually cleaner and keep dirt, bacteria and infection from re-entering the body, which can happen as you sit in dirty bath water. If you are unable to stand in the shower, invest in a shower chair to sit and hold a removable shower head.

Shower Everyday – Using a mild soap, shower with warm water, not hot water. Hot water destroys the outer most layer of skin and the "good" bacteria your body and skin needs to fight the "bad" bacteria. Shower after exercising, sweating and working with or around chemicals or smoke.

Avoid Tight Clothing – When you wear tight clothing, it can trap sweat, dirt and bacteria against the skin where it "pools" inside your hair follicles and cause folliculitis. When you choose lose-fitting clothing, you allow your skin to "breathe" and have less friction, another cause of folliculitis.

Change and Launder all Linens and Towels – When you are suffering from folliculitis, be sure to change your sheets and wash them in hot soapy water with bleach on a daily basis until the infection is cleared up. Staph infections can spread through sheets and towels and should not be shared or handled by others.

Avoid Sharing – When it comes to the prevention of folliculitis infections, sharing personal items, sports equipment or clothing is strictly off limits.

Never share combs, makeup, sleeping bags, hats, gloves, pens or pencils (some people put them behind their ear or in their hair) or anything that has touched your body.

Clean Infected Area – If a pustule opens and oozes on the skin and hair follicles nearby, it can infect that area as well and even re-infect the original hair follicle. You will need to clean the infection off your skin immediately with an antibacterial soap or an antiseptic cleanser.

Avoid Using Oils – Do not use oils on your skin because the oil, even thinner ones, can clog the hair follicle and cause surface or sweat bacteria to become trapped, causing folliculitis.

Avoid Public Hot Tubs and Swimming Pools – Public hot tubs and swimming pools can cause Hot Tube Folliculitis from dirty and improperly chemically pH balanced waters. If you cannot avoid hot tubs and swimming pools and do use these public water sources, always shower immediately after exiting the water and removing your bathing suit. Be sure to shower with a mild antibacterial soap and do not rub but pat dry with a clean towel. Wash your bathing suit in hot soapy water with bleach and do not leave it in the clothes hamper where the water can infect other clothing.

Avoid Spreading Your Infection – If you are infected, avoid spreading the bacteria to nearby skin with your razor during shaving. You could also damage the bumps and make the skin worse so it is highly recommended you avoid shaving the infected area for as long as the pustules are present. This recommendation is for anywhere on your body that is infected; shaving should be temporarily suspended. However, if you need to shave, you will need to change the blade after each shaving session. You might also look into alternative hair removal methods such as depilatory lotions or creams. Although, these home hair removing techniques are harsh and designed to be used sparingly such as one or two times a week. They could also aggregate your folliculitis infection.

Avoid Scratching/Picking/Popping – Scratching will spread the infection to the nearby follicles and you will soon have more to scratch. Picking and popping the infected bumps makes skin worse, not better. For some individuals, they cannot help themselves and the urge to pop or pick at an imperfection is overwhelming, but if this is you, you need to try as hard as you can to resist. Sometimes popping the "whitehead" pustules will only serve to bring more and more redness to a larger and larger area of your skin. Once the folliculitis in on its way to healing, picking it will not "hurry" it along and could cause more damage.

Final Thoughts

There are many individuals who are more susceptible to folliculitis outbreaks then others. And there are some individuals who may find one or two small spots of infection here or there every few years but never be that bothered by it. Folliculitis affects everyone with hair follicles and that means everyone, no matter their age, sex, socioeconomic situation, occupation or geographic home.

Prevention through diet and exercise is the first line of defense for this painful and embarrassing skin infection. When you feel good, you look good. Just remember to shower after working out. And if you do discover folliculitis, don't panic and don't pick or pop the bumps. See if you can determine the source of the infection, as well as what type, bacterial or fungal, and go from there.

If your folliculitis is too painful, too deep or doesn't seem to respond to any treatments outlined here, seek the advice of your personal physician.

Legal Notice